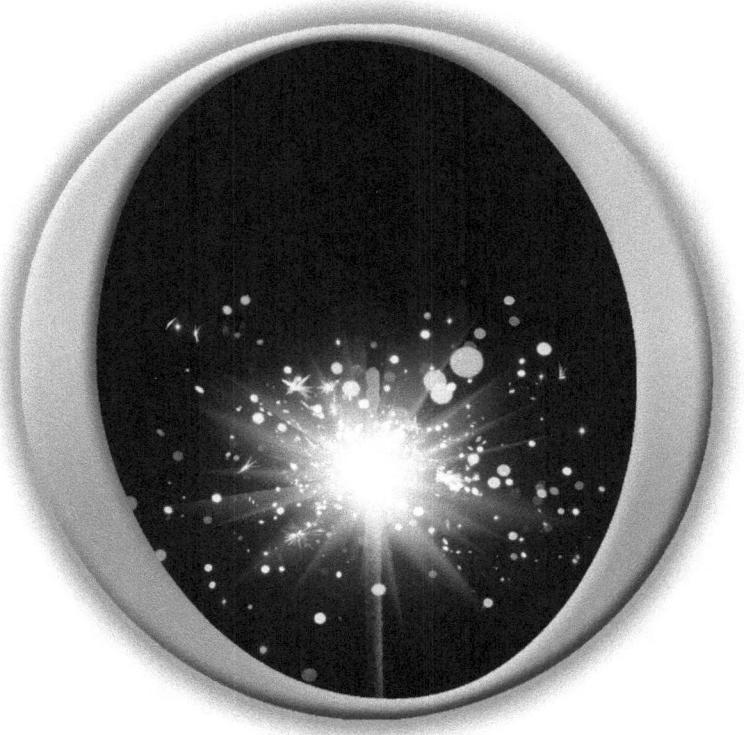

BORN IN

ORGASMIC BLISS

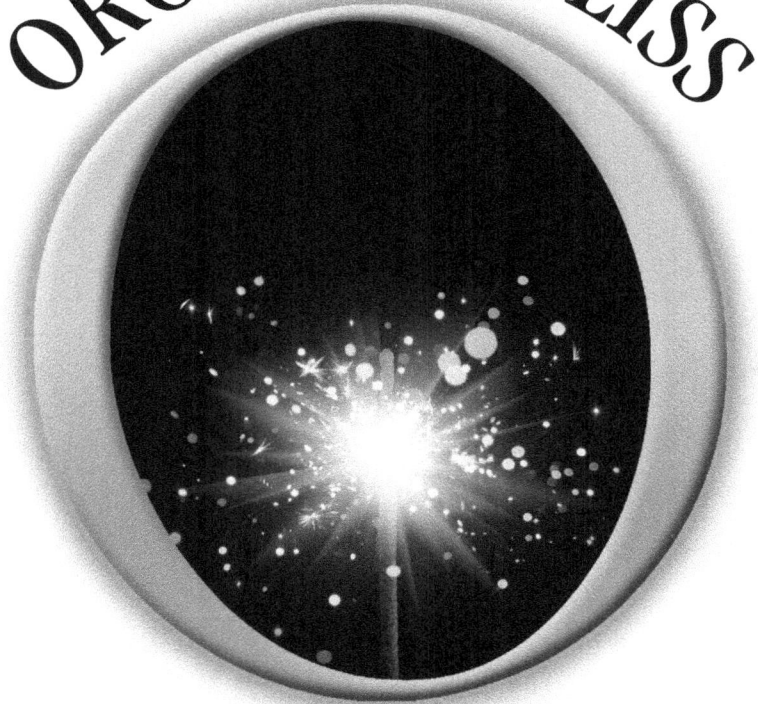

Turn Your Contractions into Expansions

Merrie P. Wycoff, Ph.D

Rosa Mystica Publishing, Colorado

Born in Orgasmic Bliss: Turn Your Contractions into Expansions
by Merrie P. Wycoff, Ph.D.

Published by:

Rosa Mystica Publishing, Colorado

Cover and Interior Design: Nick Zelinger (NZ Graphics)
Editor: Jessica Wulf
Creative Consultant: Judith Briles, (The Book Shepherd)

ISBN: 978-0-615-75781-0

Library of Congress Control Number: 2013902771

First Edition

Printed in the United States of America

Disclaimer:

I, Merrie P Wycoff, Author, am not a medical doctor. The opinions expressed and information contained in my books, videos, and websites reflect my personal experiences and ongoing investigations into childbirth, health and nutrition. The information provided in this book is designed to provide helpful information on the subjects discussed. This book is not meant to be used, nor should it be used, to diagnose or treat any medical condition nor select a course of action. For diagnosis or treatment of any medical problem, or selection of course of action, consult your own physician. The publisher and author are not responsible for any specific health or allergy needs that may require medical supervision or treatment, and are not liable for any damages or negative consequences from any treatment, action, application or preparation, to any person reading or following the information in this book. References are provided for informational purposes only and do not constitute endorsement of any books, websites or other sources,or information contained therein.

CONTENTS

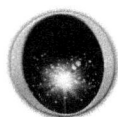

Introduction

In 1991, I was preparing to deliver my first child in Tarzana, California. I was ahead of my time. Having worked at *Entertainment Tonight* for many years, most of my pregnant friends had decided to get epidurals, or agreed to have Cesarean Sections. They explained that they didn't want to be woken up until after they had their nails done and had their hair styled. Are we so jaded that an event that usually happens naturally has to be scheduled for our convenience? When did our culture, based on instant gratification, put convenience before the well-being of a child? Somehow we forgot our connection to God and that there is god-intelligence within our unborn child. Our babies have their own astrology, destinies to fulfill, and have selected their own timing. Who are we to interfere unless there is a medical emergency? Do we change our child's destiny if we impose an inaccurate time of delivery?

When I announced that I planned to give birth naturally, my friends were appalled and asked "Why go through that much pain?" They thought I was crazy when I explained that I would do anything to bring a child into this world and give her the best chance possible. I am not a medical doctor, nor am I offering any medical advice; I am only presenting suggestions as to how I achieved two orgasmic births for both my dear daughters. People find this hard to believe, as having an 'orgasmic labor' is an oxymoron.

This book is about intimacy between you, your partner and a higher source. Our society has turned giving birth into a spectator sport with lights, cameras and action. My philosophy is that in order to create an orgasmic labor, the setting has to be intimate. No, there are no appliances necessary, nor any physical stimulation. **Orgasmic labor is NOT a sexual experience**, but an unforgettable, cosmic one.

Statistics claim that our two biggest fears are the fear of falling and loud noises. Those two fears stem directly from the birth experience. When we bear children in fear and pain, they will always have a hostile survival mentality. When we birth children in bliss, they are loving, compassionate and curious. *Born in Orgasmic Bliss* revolutionizes childbirth and explains why a bliss-filled birth is essential to welcoming in a new breed of fully integrated children.

Whether through a difficult Cesarean, epidural, or natural childbirth, there is a somatic and energetic trauma that I believe creates neurological issues around the human conscious development. My brother was pulled out by forceps and suffered from learning disabilities his entire life.

Any birth that starts out in a traumatic, frightening, constricting, or damaging condition creates later anxiety issues and hostility that plagues the entire human experience. In many ways, we never complete our birth, so how can we ever feel alive?

My goal is to introduce women to the possibility of creating a conscious birth for both you and your baby, one that will transcend and transform the whole idea that childbirth has to be painful and terrifying.

In ancient Egypt, the temple priestesses at the birthing centers would do harmonic singing at the moment of birth so the child could maintain her connection to the higher worlds from where she came. That way these beings could feel that divine connection as they entered the world, and as they left the world. They remembered how to go home.

Neurologists say we only use 5% of our brain capacity. What if we reduce or eliminate the birth trauma so that we could retain our natural psychic abilities, clairvoyance, clairsentience, clairaudience, and retro-cognitive memory of past lives? The right side of the brain could potentially be more active and balance the over-developed left brain. I believe it is our duty for women to create this evolutionary leap in consciousness to ensure that the next visionary children who are critical thinkers enter our world to help find the solutions to the problems that exist on this planet.

I understand that having an orgasm during child birth is rare. Apparently, my nurse had never seen anyone else experience bliss while giving birth either. I am living proof that what you put your mind to you can achieve.

Blessings,
Merrie P. Wycoff, Ph.D.

Birth is a rite of passage of women. Their journey should be honored, their rights should be fiercely protected, and their stories should be shared.

– Marcie Macari

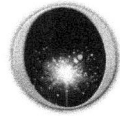

My Prophetic First Gift

I had known Jeff Wycoff for about six months before our first date, when he showed up with a beautifully wrapped present. He told me he had something special for me. As with any woman with the notion of romance floating in her head, I imagined he'd bring a bouquet of roses or Godiva chocolates.

Anyone would have guessed that his carefully wrapped thin package was a book. Poems? Fashion? Nope, it was a book about giving birth titled, *Birth Without Violence*. What kind of man would present a woman he didn't know intimately with a birthing book on their first date? Obviously, a very intuitive one, since he gave me the explanation that he understood that having children was very important to me.

I didn't give it much thought then, but two years later, after we got married we turned our attention to getting pregnant. I had to go find that book that I had shoved into some dark corner.

"Just as a woman's heart knows how and
when to pump, her lungs to inhale, and
her hand to pull back from fire, so she
knows when and how to give birth."

~ Virginia Di Orio

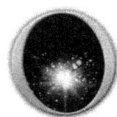

The Preparation

Society has taken a quantum leap forward in terms of teaching women that they should prepare their bodies in order to conceive and provide a nutrient-rich womb for the baby to grow. I'd spent eight years in the entertainment industry grazing off of the Craft Services tables, so my diet consisted of pizza, French fries, chocolate and orange juice. I knew that I didn't feel well but I looked thin and I thought that was all that mattered in Hollywood.

My husband had spent 18 years as a macrobiotic student of Mischio Kushi's, in Boston. His education in how food affected the body was profound. We started dating and I explained to him that he would need to own a tux because I lived a black tie dinner life. We had an amazing time, but I felt fatigued and my head was always foggy. I remember wishing that every event would be over soon so that I could go home to bed.

Candida albicans can cause infections (candidiasis or thrush) in humans and other animals, especially in immunocompromised patients.

After a while, Jeff asked me to go with him to a naturo-
pathic doctor he'd found because he suspected that he had
Candida, which is an overgrowth of yeast in the system. I
felt bad for him, and felt that I should be the supportive
girlfriend and give him comfort.

When the female doctor had taken a blood sample and
did muscle testing on him, it turned out that his blood was
incredibly healthy. He didn't have Candia at all. I was so
happy for him because the condition sounded scary. The
doctor suggested that as long as I was there I should get a
blood test and do some muscle testing too, and to my utter
surprise, my test turned out positive. Candida was attacking
my brain and nervous system. After she asked many questions,
I admitted that I had taken bags of tetracycline prescribed
by my dermatologist for adolescent acne.

All those years of heavy antibiotic use had killed off the
good intestinal flora in my digestive system. My poor diet
caused an overgrowth of yeast, which fed off of all the food I
loved and craved. My immune system was compromised, so
it was no wonder I always had a severe cough during the
colder months.

Sugar

- Check labels for lactose, sucrose, fructose and artificial sweeteners.

- Soft drinks and sugar free drinks feed Candida, too.

Dairy

- Avoid all dairy including goat and sheep milk.

- Avoid whey, buttermilk, cheese, yoghurt and cream.

Alcohol

- All alcohol stresses your organs and has a high sugar content.

Wheat, rye, barley, oats and Yeasted bread

- Gluten intolerance is on the rise.

- Corn by-products are often contaminated with fungi that is toxic to the system.

- White rice can cause glucose fluxuations.

"The human body doesn't get sick for no reason ... 90% of why people are sick, is because they eat shit."

~ Bill Maher

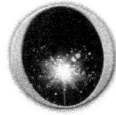

The Cleanse

I cried for days because if I cut dairy, sugar, and bread out of my diet, then what would I eat? Jeff took me back to his place and made me a bowl of Miso soup, which was a broth made from fermented soy beans. My body loved it because the soup was alkaline. I had become so acidic that the soup helped to create a balance, and felt soothing and nourishing. I remember feeling my body light up with a grid system. I asked God, "What do I have to do to keep feeling like this?" His reply was, "Give up chocolate." I pondered that—then asked, "What's my next choice?"

For the next three months I eliminated soda, ice cream, milkshakes, pizza and alcohol, and I started a simple diet of chicken, fish, brown rice and lots of vegetables and miso soup. I underwent terrible withdrawals. I cried and became irritable and I had to sleep all weekend long for three months. There were days I felt nauseous and dizzy. I went through many healing crises as I began to inch my way back to health.

Slowly though, my body underwent an amazing transformation. I'll never forget the day I looked at the trees and realized I could see the individual leaves. It was like putting on glasses for the first time. My brain and the inflammation that I had lived with since I was a teenager had vanished. My headaches disappeared and so did the exhaustion. I became more vibrant and easily lost weight. My skin was radiant. My fingers laced together without feeling swollen. My mood improved. My feet didn't itch or sweat. I felt healthier, happier, and had greater clarity. I was committed to eating right and to start taking vitamins to keep me healthy.

"To Find Health Should Be the Object of
the Doctor. Anyone Can Find Disease."

~ Andrew Taylor Still

"The doctor of the future will give no
medicine, but will interest his patient in
the care of the human frame, in diet and
in the cause and prevention of disease."

~ Thomas Edison

"After my pregnancy, I discovered
I have an allergy to yeast. Problem is,
all the food I love has yeast in it.
So I have to relearn how to cook."

~ Tia Mowry

"Women's bodies have their own
wisdom, and a system of birth refined
over 100,000 generations is not so
easily overpowered."
~ Sarah Buckley

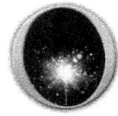

The Connection

The ancient Egyptians believed that women emit a pink light in their womb when they are pregnant, and, if one has the ability to 'see' it, it is quite amazing. I believe that babies have consciousness and are aware of what happens to the mother during their gestation. I remember being in my mother's womb and I recall an argument between my parents prior to my birth that my mother confirmed later in my life.

In my book, *Shadow of the Sun*, my paranormal historical fiction about ancient Egypt, I wrote that the protagonist, after being born, prayed "that her new mother would nourish her soul and her body in this life."

Wouldn't that be every newborn's wish? That as the parents of these blessed new babies, we would give them every opportunity to grow in a nurturing environment in order to bring out our children's greatest gifts and to guide them on their paths? I believe that is the responsibility we agree to with the children who come through us.

My first daughter appeared to me in a vision before she was born and I knew she'd be my golden-haired girl. I would talk to her mentally all the time. When my husband came home at night, he sang to her while she was still inside me. I had named her when I was 10 years old, after seeing a street sign in San Jose, California. When I said her name, it was as if the angels sang to me. That was when it dawned on me that these children who are gifted to us are angels in disguise and should be treated with respect and love, for they will one day be our teachers.

Your children are not your children.
They are the sons and daughters of Life's longing
for itself.
They come through you but not from you,
And though they are with you, yet they belong
not to you.

You may give them your love but not your thoughts.
For they have their own thoughts.
You may house their bodies but not their souls,
For their souls dwell in the house of tomorrow,
which you cannot visit, not even in your dreams.

You may strive to be like them, but seek not to make
them like you.
For life goes not backward, nor tarries with yesterday.
You are the bows from which your children as living
arrows are sent forth.

The Archer sees the mark upon the path of the
infinite, and He bends you with His might that His
arrows may go swift and far.

Let your bending in the Archer's hand be for gladness;
For even as He loves the arrow that flies, so He loves
also the bow that is stable.

Khalil Gibran

"Pregnant women! They had that weird
frisson, an aura of magic that combined
awkwardly with an earthy sense of duty.
Mundane, because they were nothing
unique on the suburban streets;
ethereal because their attention was
ever somewhere else. Whatever you said
was trivial. And they had that preciousness
which they imposed wherever they went,
compelling attention, constantly
reminding you that they carried
the future inside, its contours already
drawn, but veiled, private,
an inner secret."

~ Ruth Morgan

"A baby is something you carry inside
you for nine months, in your arms
for three years, and in your heart
til the day you die."

~ Mary Mason

"Birth is not only about making babies.
Birth is about making mothers ~ strong,
competent, capable mothers who
trust themselves and know their
inner strength."

~ Barbara Katz Rothman

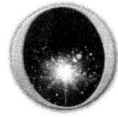

Spiritual Midwifery

Sitting in meditation one night, I received a powerful vision of Divine Mother, who told me to prepare for a great initiation. When I asked for clarification, she explained that childbirth is one of our greatest initiations into woman-hood. That by accepting this responsibility and meeting the challenge of the pain brings our consciousness to a new threshold of understanding, compassion and love. It is a gift to be able to bring life into the world, and we should be present mentally and physically to experience it.

It took me days to sort out those words. Pain? How much pain? I had never experienced real pain in my body. I had never broken a bone or hurt myself, so how could I possibly understand pain? Was it going to be so terrible that I couldn't handle it? So many of my friends were choosing Cesareans and epidurals to numb the pain of giving birth that I wondered if maybe they knew something I didn't. Fear started to well up in me. Maybe I was being ridiculous to even think about a natural birth. Who could I ask? I had been six weeks early when I was born, so my mother said that I slipped out. My OB/GYN was a man and he couldn't really understand the pain a woman would feel. In fact, he advised me to get an epidural shot.

I went to the Bodhi Tree Bookstore in Los Angeles and found the book titled *Spiritual Midwifery*, which changed the way I viewed pain. It explained that I should think of expansions rather than contractions. I should visualize the core of me opening rather than tightening. Those words altered the way I viewed giving birth. I decided to meet the pain rather than fight it.

"We have a secret in our culture,
and it's not that birth is painful.
It's that women are strong."

~ Laura Stavoe Harm

"The knowledge of how to give birth
without outside intervention lies deep
within each woman. Successful
childbirth depends on an
acceptance of the process."

~ Suzanne Arms

"If a doula were a drug, it would be unethical not to use it."
~ John H. Kennell, MD

"There is no other organ quite like the uterus. If men had such an organ they would brag about it. So should we."

~ Ina May Gaskin

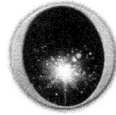

Finding a Spiritual Midwife

It became my quest to find a Doula, or Midwife, and when I looked in the phonebook there weren't many. I called one and we decided to meet. I was seven months along and she reassured me that what I was feeling was normal. She said, like other women had, that the pain of childbirth is a pain that passes because of the joy it brings when you see your new baby. That made sense, but I still felt anxious.

When a woman is giving birth, she has sorrow because her hour has come, but when she has delivered the baby, she no longer remembers the anguish, for joy that a human being has been born into the world. – John 16:21

The midwife taught me breathing exercises and visualization techniques along with stretching exercises after I told her that I didn't want an episiotomy or to have my perineum cut in order to give birth. Yeah, call me crazy, but I was determined to do it the old-fashioned way.

After reading *Spiritual Midwifery*, I discovered a new way of giving birth in water that was being done in France. I got a video tape of a woman giving birth in the ocean and watched that new baby swim to the surface. Although I lived near Malibu, I didn't want to stand in the Pacific Ocean next to surfers and swimmers while grunting out a child. The next option was to have a home birth in my huge bathtub. My husband agreed to it as long as we had a backup plan to get to a hospital should something go wrong. I tried to discuss this with my OB/GYN but he thought it was ridiculous.

"Muscles send messages to each other. Clenched fists, a tight mouth, a furrowed brow, all send signals to the birth-passage muscles, the very ones that need to be loosened. Opening up to relax these upper-body parts relaxes the lower ones."

~ William and Martha Sears

**"If you lay down, the baby will
never come out!"**
~ Native American saying

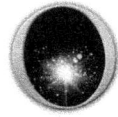

Being Your Own Advocate

The World Health Organization says that there isn't any medical reason for a Cesarean birthrate higher than 15 percent. Yet, here in Colorado the C-Section rate is 24 percent. The *New York Times* reported that in 2007, the Caesarean Section rate had reached 32 percent in the United States, which was the country's all time high. A C-Section was the most common operation in the hospitals in the USA.

Critics oppose Caesareans and claim the operation is performed way more than necessary and that this operation exposes both the mothers and the babies to risks because it is considered major surgery. When this procedure is performed to save the life of a mother or a child and prevent injury or death, then of course it is necessary. But all operations have a greater chance of infection and hemorrhaging. Currently, one in three women are receiving C-Sections versus vaginal births, and that also increases the possibility of post-partum depression.

If there is increased chance of side effects, why would doctors encourage women to have a C-Section? According to the Healthcare Research and Quality, a vaginal birth without complications in a Colorado hospital averages about $9,000, while a C-Section birth without complications averages about $15,755. Would this necessarily influence doctors to recommend the later procedure?

Chances are that when you go into labor and check into your hospital, you'll find that your health care providers have a pool of network obstetricians on call. A mother might not 'get' the doctor with whom she has been working; if she had planned on having a natural birth without an epidural or induced labor, then she also might not 'get' the birth she had envisioned.

When labor is induced the contractions intensify and an epideral will likely be administered.

Active labor begins at 1-2 centimeters. Unless you have a fever, or you or the baby are in distress, it would be wise to wait until active labor begins for all normal births before you go to the hospital. The best way to avoid a medical intervention for a normal birth is to use a midwife or doula as a guide.

"The power and intensity of your
contractions cannot be stronger
than you, because it is you."

~ Unknown

"There is no way out of the experience except through it, because it is not really your experience at all but the baby's. Your body is the child's instrument of birth."

~ Penelope Leach

"Only with trust, faith, and support
can the woman allow the birth experience
to enlighten and empower her."
~ Claudia Lowe

"Attending births is like growing roses. You have to marvel at the ones that just open up and bloom at the first kiss of the sun but you wouldn't dream of pulling open the petals of the tightly closed buds and forcing them to blossom to your time line."

~ Gloria Lemay

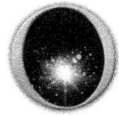

Clearing the Past

When I was about two weeks away from my due date, I went to my midwife for an exam, and she explained that the baby had not dropped yet. She told me that I still had fear in me from a previous life. What? Now I was responsible for every past life in which I gave birth? How fair was that? Who could even remember back that far? Well, what was my option? I knew I had my work cut out for me.

I meditated that night and asked God to show me the way. What old fear did I need to face? What was keeping my daughter from turning? Images soon flashed through my mind, and I saw myself in the Gobi Desert with a man who in that lifetime was my husband. He wanted and needed a son to succeed him. When I gave birth by myself and produced a girl, he left us to die.

I started to sob. I knew I was having a girl. Did this old fear still have a hold on me? The pain and fear of rejection and abandonment were overwhelming to me. But I stayed with the image until I felt a clearing in my body. I asked for any other images from the past that was hindering my daughter's willingness to turn, and the energy was all clear.

Strangely enough, she turned the next morning and I thought we were good to go. Now, my only concern was that the midwife could make the hour-plus drive from Pasadena to the San Fernando Valley without traffic. Hey, I thought, why couldn't I just ask my daughter to start labor around 2 am? Then I could notify the midwife before all the traffic. I know willing labor to start sounds nuts, but then, from the beginning I hadn't handled this pregnancy in the traditional way. I did and still do believe these tiny beings choose their own time of birth.

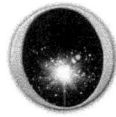

Be Flexible

I waited patiently until August rolled around, then I was ready to get this over with. Now I was 1 week past my due date. Being pregnant in the heat of summer was hard. Every night I suggested that 2 am would be a great time to get started. But kids have minds of their own and their own contracts with God. I would have to trust that a Divine Intelligence was taking care of all this.

Another week passed and I started to get anxious again. I said tonight would be really good because my husband didn't have to work the next day. Sure enough, the first stab of pain hit me and woke me up. I glanced at the clock; it was 2 am. I had to laugh, and I thanked my daughter for being so thoughtful. I slept a bit more, and by 6am, I started to feel the contractions come more consistently. I called the midwife and she said she'd leave in an hour.

By 8:30 am she arrived, and my husband had filled up the tub and got out the plastic sheets and extra towels for a water home birth. He had been massaging my back and neck. I was so pleased because the contractions, while a bit uncomfortable, were certainly manageable.

When the midwife used her stethoscope to listen to the heartbeat, she looked alarmed. "What's wrong?" I asked.

"She has an A-rhythm," she replied as she palpated my abdomen. The midwife explained that an A-rhythm was Arrhythmia, an inconsistent heartbeat. There could something be wrong with the child's heart, or she could just be holding on to the umbilical cord, but either way, the midwife no longer felt comfortable with a homebirth and suggested an emergency C-Section.

We hurriedly threw things in the overnight bag and jumped in the car. It was nonstop traffic to Tarzana Hospital on the busy Los Angeles 405 Highway. I teared up at the thought that after all my careful planning I would have to have a C-Section anyway. I admit I felt like a failure. This would be a nightmare. Everything I had hoped to avoid was happening to me. My husband held my hand and told me to not worry, that either way my health and the health of our baby took precedence over the dream of a natural birth.

The entire way to the hospital I asked God for direction and I kept hearing Do Not Worry … ALL Will Be Well. We checked in and they rushed me to the Emergency Ward while my husband had to stay back and sign papers. What I didn't know was that he had refused to sign anything until I was checked out by a doctor. My OB/GYN said that the only way he would downgrade the C-Section to a natural birth or direct us to a private birthing room was if the A-rhythm stopped.

"Life is tough enough without having someone kick you from the inside."

~ Rita Rudner

"People are giving birth underwater now. They say it's less traumatic for the baby because it's in water. But certainly more traumatic for the other people in the pool."

~ Elayne Boosler

"Because they've either conveniently forgotten with time or they're trying to be supportive, most mothers won't tell you how hard pregnancy (and then childbirth) can be. Let me tell you, it is. It's brutal sometimes! But, if I did it, ANYONE can do it. I mean, I always knew I was meant to do something really BIG in life, and now I know that this was it. Screw winning an Academy Award someday ... I GAVE BIRTH."

~ Jenny McCarthy

"I'm not interested in being
Wonder Woman in the delivery room.
Give me drugs."
~ Madonna

"I am not finding pregnancy much
of a joy. I am afraid of childbirth,
but I am afraid I can't find a way
of avoiding it."

~ Brigitte Bardot

"Giving birth should be your greatest
achievement not your greatest fear. "

~ Jane Weideman

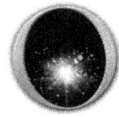

Translating the Pain

I felt a deep connection with my baby. Recalling back to when she had hiccups and my belly jiggled, I would think soothing thoughts to her and the hiccups would disappear. Now, I 'thought' to my daughter that I intended to have a beautiful natural birth and that I needed her help. I asked her to let go of the umbilical cord. I was not surprised when she did. The A-rhythm stopped and they downgraded the emergency C-Section to a natural birth with monitors.

I still ended up being hooked to machines to check her heartbeat, but at least I was in a private room. They allowed my midwife to attend the birth. My husband rubbed my shoulders and looked into my eyes. He told me he loved me, over and over again. He gave me his love and support, a deep feeling of trust that I could do this and that he was there for me. I demanded that he continue this for hours, even though he was starving. I wouldn't let him leave to get a sandwich. Call me crazy, but I was in pain, and I felt that since I couldn't eat, why should he?

When the contractions began to intensify, my fear started to nibble at me. Questions flooded my mind. What if I became too exhausted to push? How much longer can this go on? What if it gets worse? I had to calm myself. With every contraction, I made a choice that I would turn the tightening into an expansion. I envisioned my womb opening up to release my child. A feeling of peace washed over me. I knew that God wouldn't give me more than I could handle.

I had heard there is only a fine line between pain and pleasure, and I wondered where that line was. What was my pain threshold? I knew that when endorphins kicked in, pain trauma could be numbed to protect the patient.

Couldn't that apply to childbirth? The expansions I was feeling weren't intolerable. I was determined to explore this and go *into* the pain rather than fight against it or feel anxiety about it.

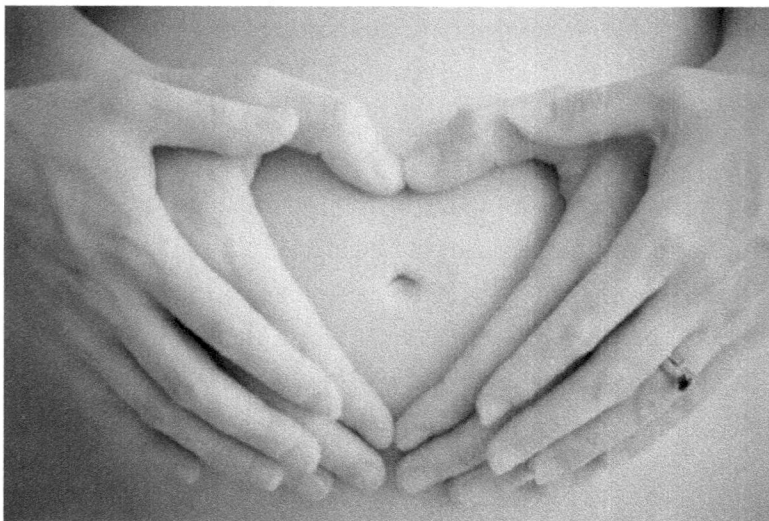

With the next expansion I opened to the pain. The word 'translate' came into my mind. I allowed the pain to feel good and productive versus feeling overwhelmed by it. I became empowered and knew that I could take control of my body; a switch flipped in my mind. It started slowly but an orgasm began to build. My body knew how to numb the pain and feel pleasure by the intensity of expansions. I started moaning softly and feeling that utter state of bliss. I was about 9 cm and nearing time to push.

The nurse walked in and looked embarrassed. She asked, "Do you want some pain meds?" I said, "What could be better than a 45-minute orgasm? No pain meds would be better than this."

She said that in all her years she had never seen anything like this and that it was way too intimate for her, so she left. My midwife told me to just enjoy it because I was almost there. My daughter was born an hour later. My husband was able to deliver her and place her on my stomach. My daughter's eyes were open and she was fully present. She nursed within a few minutes and I held and loved her from the moment she was born. We refused to allow anyone to take her away.

My cranial sacral therapist arrived and did a session on my daughter. My naturopath also adjusted her cranium to relieve any birth trauma and balance her brain and nervous system.

My oldest daughter still remembers her birth; she remembers what I was wearing, and the car we got into the next day. During her early years she could write forward and backwards in a mirror image. She is fluent in languages and feels safe in the world.

- Pull the curtains. Darken the room.

- Spray your favorite fragrance.

- Have your ipod playing classical or new age music— something soothing without an intense beat.

- Make eye contact with your partner.

- Receive massages on your neck and shoulders and lower back.

- Wear colorful fuzzy socks.

- Have your partner tell you that they love you and that you are doing great.

- Think of expansions rather than contractions.

- Move into the pain and ride above it, wait until the endorphins kick in and the pain is numbed.

- Use the pain as a stimulant to move into orgasm.

- Keep the experience intimate. Unless you are confident, it is hard to share this with a room full of family and friends.

- Sip spoonfuls of raspberry tea to ease labor.

- Take a few drops of Rescue Remedy homeopathic if you feel panic coming on.

- Remember to Breathe!

"Maybe I was just lucky, but I had the
best pregnancy, and I loved giving birth.
It was just the most amazing thing,
so surreal but so real."

~ Ashlee Simpson

"I think one of the best things we could do would be to help women/parents/families discover their own birth power, from within themselves. And to let them know it's always been there, they just needed to tap into it."

~ Karl Menninger

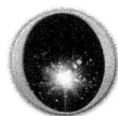

A Husband's Perspective

The contractions were now coming every 15 minutes. The doctor checked my wife's dilation. "Not long," he said and left. I leaned over and asked her, "What can I do for you?" She said, "Tell me you love me, and don't stop until she arrives." So rhythmically I repeated those three words. "I LOVE YOU, I LOVE YOU."

Something magical happened. Merrie's eyes slowly closed, her faced relaxed. This look washed over her face, one of bliss. I once believed that the experience of giving birth was of overwhelming pain, screaming, and pain medication. This was truly the opposite for us. Merrie decided she was going to take control of this birth; this was going to be an orgasmic experience, not a painful one. The more I said those three words, the more blissful she became.

It was something powerful to behold. My wife is a soft, kind and gentle woman, yet it was as if she was channeling this incredible strength, such warmth and softness at the same time. The Gods had given her the power of Zeus, harnessing those lightning bolts mixed with Hera's ability to procreate.

We had agreed long before that I would deliver the baby, but I couldn't stop saying those three words … I didn't want to. My heart had become one with hers. Without hesitation

I moved to the end of the bed and delivered our first daughter. The baby slid out into my arms, with her hand pulling her hair. She opened her eyes and I could tell that she knew who I was. I carried her to her mother's breast where she, with all the contentment in her little body, began to suckle. I stood over the two of them still lost in those three words.

To this day, I have never seen anything so beautiful, especially my wife. You have heard the expression, "She looked like an angel." Well, my wife *was an angel,* and I will never forget the power of those three words.

Merrie ... I love you!

~ Jeff Wycoff

"Making a decision to have a child—it's
momentous. It is to decide forever to
have your heart go walking around
outside your body."

~ Elizabeth Stone

"The child suddenly finds itself liberated
from an unendurable captivity…and
weeps! This also happens to prisoners
who are suddenly set free."

~ LeBoyer

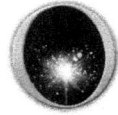

Birth Without Violence

For my second daughter's birth, we went to the hospital and got the natural birth room. I was able to walk around the room, take a shower and relax. Again, I had another hour-long orgasm during the contraction period, and when it came time to deliver, we asked to squat and use a birthing bar. The bar was in the janitor's closet because no one had ever used it before.

My husband gave me shoulder and lower back massages. We played music by Kitaro, burned incense, and had the lights dimmed. Everyone was asked to use soft voices. I used the method of Frederick LeBoyer, an obstetrician who delivered more than 10,000 babies. His book, *Birth Without Violence*, advocates for the use of simple techniques to reduce birth trauma and to assist the newborn to begin a life without 'pain, confusion and fear.' His theory is that the womb is a warm, constricted, quiet place and the baby typically comes into a room with blaring lights, chaotic voices barking orders, and the air is cold and harsh; those sensory shocks alter a child's impression of the world. By softening all that, the child enters with more ease and grace. And because the fetus's brain emerges from its heart, we should assist by cultivating loving thoughts within the child's brain. To begin, we cultivate love within the mother's heart.

My second daughter's eyes were open and she recognized her father's voice when he said, "Don't worry, Daddy is here." She visibly sighed and relaxed and began to suckle immediately. I massaged her back and talked to her. Again, we wouldn't allow the nurses to take her away from us.

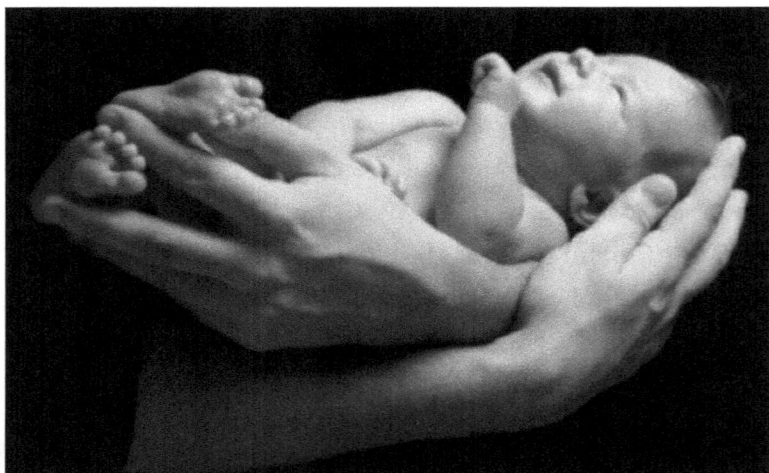

"Rain, after all, is only rain;
it is not bad weather. So also,
pain is only pain; unless we resist it,
then it becomes torment."
~ I Ching

**"You're braver than you believe.
Stronger than you seem.
And smarter than you think."**
~ Christopher Robin in *Pooh's Grand Adventure*

"The spiritual quality of earth:
eternally pregnant and containing
in its fertility the unwritten cipher
of cosmic lore."

~ Lady Frieda Harris

"When you change the way you view
birth, the way you birth will change."

~ Marie Mongan

"Let go. Trust that women have done
this for eons. Trust that you have
the power to will your flower to
unfurl and release the fruit."

~ Merrie P. Wycoff

10 Reasons To Breast Feed

1) Increases your child's IQ by 7 point average

2) Risk of SIDS-related death is reduced

3) Reduces the risk of the baby's allergic reaction

4) Burns calories for Mom, up to 500 per day

5) Reduces the risk of postpartum hemorrhage

6) Baby is less likely to develop type 1 Diabetes

7) Mom's risk of breast cancer diminishes

8) Child is less likely to suffer from ear infections

9) Signals Mom to lose baby fat naturally

10) It is convenient

Recommended by the American Academy of Pediatrics (AAP)

"There are three reasons for
breast-feeding: the milk is always
at the right temperature;
it comes in attractive containers;
and the cat can't get it."

~ Irena Chalmers

"Breast milk contains virtually all of
the nutrients that an infant needs except
for Vitamin D ... That's because
infants weren't designed to swallow
the vitamin D, they were designed to
have sun on their skin."

~ Dr. Mercola

"It's not natural for humans to drink cow's milk. Humans milk is for humans. Cow's milk is for calves. You have no more need of cow's milk than you do rats milk, horses milk or elephant's milk. Cow's milk is a high fat fluid exquisitely designed to turn a 65 lb baby calf into a 400 lb cow. That's what cow's milk is for!"

~ Dr. Michael Klaper, MD

"It is not only that we want to bring about an easy labor, without risking injury to the mother or the child; we must go further. We must understand that childbirth is fundamentally a spiritual, as well as a physical, achievement. The birth of a child is the ultimate perfection of human love."
~ Dr. Grantly Dick-Read, 1953

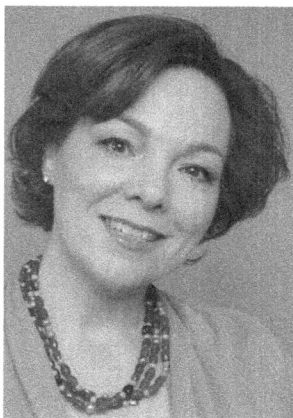

About the Author

At the age of ten, while on a school field trip to a local museum, Merrie P. Wycoff saw a colossal statue of Pharaoh Ahkenaten. She was instantly mesmerized, and so was born her passion for Egypt, its history, and its ancient people. That passion has stayed with her from her growing-up years through today, fueled by her long-ago vow to write Akhenaten's story. Now, with the publication of *Shadow of the Sun*, she has fulfilled that vow.

In addition to a B.A in Public Relations, an M.A. in Metaphysical Studies, and a Ph.D. in Comparative Religions, Merrie is in the process of finishing her Egyptology degree with the University of Manchester in Great Britain.

Having worked at *Entertainment Tonight* for six years as a Segment Producer, Merrie then used those skills to create an infomercial company with her husband and launch *Zap! The Professional Restorer.*

Merrie resides in Colorado, close to the majesty and the magic of the Rocky Mountains. There she follows her triple calling as a Vibrational Healer, a writer, and a speaker. *Shadow of the Sun* is her first novel. She founded WOMBS -Women's Orgasmic Mindful Birth Sisterhood.

Born in Orgasmic Bliss
Facebook: WOMBSisterhood
Twitter: OrgasmicBirth4U
Web site: BornInOrgasmicBliss.com

What I fear about childbirth:

_____

_____

_____

_____

_____

_____

_____

_____

_____

_____

_____

_____

_____

_____

_____

_____

How was I born?:

_____

_____

_____

_____

_____

_____

_____

_____

_____

_____

_____

_____

_____

_____

www.ingramcontent.com/pod-product-compliance
Lightning Source LLC
Chambersburg PA
CBHW070911280326
41934CB00008B/1674